MITCHELL LEY

FIBROMYALGIA UNVEILED: A Complete Guide Treatment To Navigating the Landscape of Chronic Pain, Insights, and Hope.

Copyright ©2023 MITCHELL LEY All rights reserved. No part of this publication may be reproduced, distributed, or transmitted in any form or by any means, including photocopying, recording, or other electronic or mechanical methods, without the prior written permission of the publisher, except in the case of brief quotations embodied in critical reviews and certain other non-commercial uses permitted by copyright law.

Table of Contents

INTRODUCTION

Fibromyalgia is a medical condition characterized by widespread musculoskeletal pain, fatigue, sleep disturbances, and tenderness in localized areas. It is considered a chronic disorder that often coexists with other conditions such as irritable bowel syndrome (IBS), tension headaches, temporomandibular joint disorders, anxiety, and depression.

Key features of fibromyalgia include:

Pain: The pain associated with fibromyalgia is typically widespread and affects both sides of the body, above and below the waist. It is often described as a constant dull ache that lasts for at least three months.

Tender Points: These are specific points on the body that are particularly sensitive to pressure. There are 18 designated tender points associated with fibromyalgia.

Fatigue: People with fibromyalgia often experience persistent fatigue, even after a full night's sleep. Sleep disturbances, such as insomnia or non-restorative sleep, are common in individuals with fibromyalgia.

Cognitive Difficulties: Often referred to as "fibro fog," individuals with fibromyalgia may experience difficulties with concentration, memory, and overall cognitive function.

The exact cause of fibromyalgia is not well understood, but it is believed to involve a combination of genetic, environmental, and psychological factors. It is more common in women than in men, and it typically manifests between the ages of 30 and 60.

Diagnosing fibromyalgia can be challenging, as there is no specific test for it. Healthcare providers often rely on a combination of clinical symptoms and a physical examination, including the presence of tender points, to make a diagnosis. Other conditions with similar symptoms need to be ruled out.

Treatment for fibromyalgia is usually multidisciplinary and may include medications, physical therapy, exercise, stress management, and lifestyle changes. It's important for individuals with fibromyalgia to work closely with their healthcare providers to develop a personalized treatment plan.

If you suspect you have fibromyalgia or are experiencing symptoms, it's essential to consult with a healthcare professional for a proper evaluation and diagnosis.

SYMPTOMS

Widespread Pain

- **Description:** The hallmark symptom of fibromyalgia is chronic, widespread pain that affects both sides of the body and is present above and below the waist. It often involves muscles, ligaments, and tendons.

- **Characteristics:** The pain is often described as a constant dull ache, but it can vary in intensity. It may be exacerbated by factors such as weather changes, stress, or physical activity.

Tender Points

- **Description:** Fibromyalgia is associated with specific tender points on the body. These points are areas that are particularly sensitive to pressure.

- **Location:** There are 18 designated tender points, including the back of the head, neck, chest, elbows, hips, and knees. To be diagnosed with fibromyalgia, a person typically needs to have pain in at least 11 of these points.

Fatigue

- **Description:** Persistent fatigue is common in individuals with fibromyalgia, regardless of how much sleep they get. Sleep is often disrupted by pain or other symptoms.
- **Impact:** The fatigue can be overwhelming and may interfere with daily activities and work.

Sleep Disturbances

- *Description:* Many people with fibromyalgia experience sleep disturbances, such as difficulty falling asleep, staying asleep, or achieving restorative sleep.
- *Consequences:* Poor sleep can exacerbate other symptoms, including fatigue and cognitive difficulties.

Cognitive Difficulties ("Fibro Fog")

- *Description:* Individuals with fibromyalgia often report cognitive difficulties, commonly referred to as "fibro fog."
- *Symptoms:* This may include problems with concentration, memory, and the ability to focus on mental tasks.

Other Symptoms

- ***Headaches:*** Tension headaches and migraines are common in individuals with fibromyalgia.
- ***Irritable Bowel Syndrome (IBS):*** Many people with fibromyalgia also experience digestive issues, such as abdominal pain, bloating, and changes in bowel habits.
- ***Joint Pain:*** While fibromyalgia primarily involves soft tissues, some individuals may also experience joint pain.

Sensitivity to Stimuli

- ***Sensory Sensitivities:*** Increased sensitivity to light, noise, and temperature changes is not uncommon in fibromyalgia.
- ***Skin Sensitivity:*** Some individuals may also have heightened sensitivity to touch.

It's important to note that fibromyalgia symptoms can vary from person to person, and the severity of symptoms can fluctuate over time. Additionally, fibromyalgia symptoms can overlap with those of other conditions, which is why a comprehensive medical evaluation is necessary for an accurate diagnosis. If you suspect you may have fibromyalgia or are experiencing symptoms, it's essential to consult with a healthcare professional for proper evaluation and guidance.

DIAGNOSIS

Diagnosing fibromyalgia can be challenging because there is no specific test or imaging study that can definitively confirm its presence. Instead, healthcare providers rely on a combination of clinical evaluation, medical history, and the exclusion of other conditions with similar symptoms. Here are key aspects of the diagnosis process:

Clinical Evaluation

- *Medical History:* A detailed discussion of the patient's medical history, including the nature, duration, and severity of symptoms, is crucial. It helps identify patterns and rule out other possible causes of the symptoms.

- *Physical Examination:* The healthcare provider may conduct a physical examination to check for the characteristic tender points associated with fibromyalgia. Diagnosis often involves the presence of pain in at least 11 out of 18 designated tender points.

Exclusion of Other Conditions

- *Laboratory Tests:* Blood tests and other laboratory studies may be ordered to rule out conditions with similar symptoms, such as rheumatoid arthritis, lupus, and thyroid disorders.

- *Imaging Studies:* X-rays and other imaging studies may be conducted to rule out structural abnormalities or joint disorders.

Meeting Diagnostic Criteria

Fibromyalgia Criteria: Diagnosis is often based on criteria established by organizations such as the American College of Rheumatology (ACR). The ACR criteria include widespread pain lasting for at least three months and the presence of tender points. However, the tender point examination is not always required for diagnosis.

Symptom Severity and Impact

- *Assessment of Symptoms:* Healthcare providers assess the severity and impact of symptoms on the patient's daily life, including the level of pain, fatigue, and cognitive difficulties.

- ***Quality of Life:*** Understanding how fibromyalgia affects the patient's overall well-being is an essential component of the diagnosis.

Collaboration with Specialists

- ***Rheumatologists:*** While many healthcare providers, including primary care physicians, can diagnose and manage fibromyalgia, some patients may be referred to rheumatologists, especially when there is uncertainty about the diagnosis or if additional rheumatic conditions need to be ruled out.

- ***Multidisciplinary Approach:*** Fibromyalgia is often managed with a multidisciplinary approach that may involve rheumatologists, pain specialists, physical therapists, and mental health professionals.

It's important to note that the diagnosis of fibromyalgia is a clinical one, and healthcare providers consider a combination of factors to make an informed decision. Additionally, ongoing communication between the patient and their healthcare team is crucial for managing symptoms and adjusting the treatment plan as needed. If you suspect you have fibromyalgia or are experiencing symptoms, it's essential to consult with a healthcare professional for a thorough evaluation and diagnosis.

CAUSES AND RISK FACTORS

The exact causes of fibromyalgia are not fully understood, and it is likely that a combination of factors contributes to the development of the condition. Here are some potential causes and risk factors associated with fibromyalgia:

Genetic Factors

There appears to be a genetic component to fibromyalgia. Individuals with a family history of the condition may be at a higher risk.

Physical Trauma or Injury

Physical trauma, such as car accidents or repetitive injuries, may trigger the onset of fibromyalgia symptoms in some individuals.

Infections

Certain infections or illnesses may act as triggers for fibromyalgia in susceptible individuals. These can include viral or bacterial infections.

Stress

Physical or emotional stress may play a role in the development or exacerbation of fibromyalgia symptoms. Chronic stress can contribute to the amplification of pain and other symptoms.

Hormonal Factors

Changes in hormonal levels, particularly in women, may influence the development or severity of fibromyalgia. For example, hormonal fluctuations during the menstrual cycle or hormonal changes associated with menopause can impact symptoms.

Sleep Disturbances

Disturbed sleep patterns, such as insomnia or disruptions in the sleep cycle, are common in individuals with fibromyalgia. Some researchers believe that sleep disturbances may contribute to the development of fibromyalgia, while others consider them a consequence of the condition.

Neurochemical Imbalances

Imbalances in neurotransmitters, such as serotonin, norepinephrine, and dopamine, have been observed in individuals with fibromyalgia. These imbalances may contribute to the heightened perception of pain.

Autoimmune Factors

While fibromyalgia is not considered an autoimmune disorder, there is ongoing research exploring potential connections between fibromyalgia and autoimmune processes.

Other Health Conditions

Fibromyalgia often coexists with other health conditions, such as irritable bowel syndrome (IBS), rheumatoid arthritis, and systemic lupus erythematosus. Having these conditions may increase the risk of developing fibromyalgia.

Gender and Age

Fibromyalgia is more common in women than in men, and it most frequently occurs in individuals between the ages of 30 and 60. However, it can affect people of any age, including children.

It's important to note that while these factors may contribute to the development of fibromyalgia, the condition is complex, and individual experiences can vary widely. Additionally, some people may develop fibromyalgia without any clear predisposing factors.

Research into the causes and risk factors of fibromyalgia is ongoing, and a better understanding of these factors may contribute to improved diagnostic and treatment approaches in the future. If you have concerns about fibromyalgia or are experiencing symptoms, consulting with a healthcare professional is crucial for a thorough evaluation.

TREATMENT OPTIONS

The treatment of fibromyalgia typically involves a multidisciplinary approach that addresses the various symptoms and aspects of the condition. It's important to note that there is no cure for fibromyalgia, but treatment strategies aim to manage symptoms and improve overall quality of life. Here are common treatment options:

Medications

- **Pain Relievers:** Over-the-counter pain relievers, such as acetaminophen, may be recommended.

- **Nonsteroidal Anti-Inflammatory Drugs (NSAIDs):** NSAIDs like ibuprofen can help reduce inflammation and alleviate pain.

- **Antidepressants:** Certain antidepressant medications, such as amitriptyline, duloxetine, and milnacipran, may be prescribed to help manage pain and improve sleep.

- **Anticonvulsants:** Medications like gabapentin or pregabalin, which are commonly used to treat seizures, can be effective in reducing pain.

Physical Therapy

- **Exercise Programs:** Tailored exercise programs, including aerobic exercises, strength training, and flexibility exercises, can help improve muscle strength, reduce pain, and enhance overall well-being.
- **Physical Modalities:** Techniques such as heat therapy, cold therapy, and massage may provide relief from pain and muscle stiffness.
- **Education:** Physical therapists often educate individuals about proper body mechanics and pacing activities to prevent exacerbation of symptoms.

Cognitive-Behavioral Therapy (CBT)

- **Cognitive Restructuring:** CBT helps individuals identify and change negative thought patterns related to pain and other symptoms.
- **Behavioral Techniques:** Techniques such as relaxation training and stress management can be beneficial in managing fibromyalgia symptoms.

Lifestyle and Self-Care

- **Sleep Hygiene:** Establishing good sleep habits, such as maintaining a regular sleep schedule and creating a comfortable sleep environment, can help improve sleep quality.

- **Stress Management:** Techniques such as meditation, deep breathing exercises, and mindfulness can help manage stress and reduce symptom severity.

- **Balanced Diet:** A well-balanced diet with an emphasis on nutrient-rich foods can contribute to overall health.

Medication Management

- **Careful Medication Use:** Healthcare providers work with individuals to carefully manage medications, adjusting dosages or changing prescriptions as needed.

- **Monitoring Side Effects:** Regular monitoring of medication side effects and effectiveness is essential for optimizing treatment.

Alternative Therapies

- **Acupuncture:** Some individuals find relief from fibromyalgia symptoms through acupuncture.

- **Yoga and Tai Chi:** These mind-body practices can help improve flexibility, balance, and reduce stress.

Supportive Therapies

- **Support Groups:** Participating in support groups or counseling can provide emotional support and practical coping strategies.

- **Occupational Therapy:** Occupational therapists can help individuals adapt to daily activities and reduce strain on the body.

Pharmacological Advances

Ongoing Research: Researchers are exploring new medications and treatment approaches for fibromyalgia, and ongoing clinical trials may lead to advancements in treatment.

Treatment plans are often individualized, and what works for one person may not work for another. It's crucial for individuals with fibromyalgia to work closely with their healthcare providers to develop a comprehensive and personalized treatment approach. Regular communication, lifestyle adjustments, and ongoing self-care are key components of managing fibromyalgia effectively. If you suspect you have fibromyalgia or are experiencing symptoms, consult with a healthcare professional for a thorough

evaluation and guidance on appropriate treatment options.

LIFESTYLE AND HOME REMEDIES

Lifestyle and home remedies play a crucial role in managing fibromyalgia symptoms. While there is no one-size-fits-all approach, adopting healthy habits and making certain lifestyle adjustments can contribute to improved well-being. Here are some lifestyle and home remedies for individuals with fibromyalgia:

Establishing a Regular Sleep Routine

- Maintain a consistent sleep schedule by going to bed and waking up at the same time each day.
- Create a comfortable sleep environment, ensuring the bedroom is dark, quiet, and cool.
- Limit caffeine and stimulant intake, especially in the hours leading up to bedtime.

Regular Exercise

- Engage in low-impact exercises regularly, such as walking, swimming, or cycling.
- Incorporate flexibility exercises and gentle stretching to improve joint mobility.

- Gradually increase the intensity and duration of exercise, tailored to individual capabilities.

Stress Management

- Practice relaxation techniques, such as deep breathing, meditation, or progressive muscle relaxation.
- Identify and address sources of stress in daily life, employing strategies to cope with stressors effectively.

Balanced Diet

- Aim for a well-balanced diet rich in fruits, vegetables, whole grains, and lean proteins.
- Stay hydrated by drinking an adequate amount of water throughout the day.
- Consider consulting a registered dietitian to explore dietary modifications that may benefit symptom management.

Pacing Activities

- Break tasks into smaller, manageable segments to avoid overexertion.

- Prioritize tasks and focus on essential activities, allowing for periods of rest and recovery.
- Listen to the body's signals and adjust activity levels accordingly.

Heat and Cold Therapy

- Apply heat packs or warm compresses to areas of pain or stiffness to relax muscles.
- Use cold packs to reduce inflammation and numb localized areas of pain.
- Experiment with both heat and cold therapy to determine which provides the most relief.

Massage and Self-Massage Techniques

- Regular massages from a qualified therapist may help reduce muscle tension and pain.
- Learn and practice self-massage techniques using tools such as foam rollers or massage balls.

Mind-Body Practices

- Explore mind-body practices like yoga or tai chi to improve flexibility, balance, and mindfulness.

- Mindfulness meditation can help manage stress and enhance overall well-being.

Supportive Footwear and Ergonomics

- Choose comfortable, supportive footwear to reduce strain on joints.
- Evaluate and optimize workspaces and daily activities for ergonomic comfort.

Stay Connected

- Maintain social connections to prevent isolation and foster emotional well-being.
- Join fibromyalgia support groups, either in-person or online, to share experiences and coping strategies.

Hydrotherapy

- Warm baths or showers can provide relaxation and relief from muscle pain.
- Hydrotherapy, such as aquatic exercise in a heated pool, may be beneficial.

It's important for individuals with fibromyalgia to work collaboratively with their healthcare providers to develop a personalized approach to lifestyle and home remedies. Monitoring the effects of these strategies and making adjustments as needed is key to managing symptoms effectively. If you have specific concerns or questions, it's advisable to consult with your healthcare team for guidance tailored to your individual needs.

COMORBID CONDITIONS

Fibromyalgia often coexists with other health conditions, a phenomenon known as comorbidity. Managing these comorbid conditions is an important aspect of the overall care for individuals with fibromyalgia. Here are some common comorbid conditions associated with fibromyalgia:

Irritable Bowel Syndrome (IBS)

- **Description:** IBS is a gastrointestinal disorder characterized by abdominal pain, bloating, and changes in bowel habits.
- **Connection:** Many individuals with fibromyalgia also experience symptoms of IBS, and the two conditions often occur together.

Migraines and Headaches

- **Description:** Individuals with fibromyalgia may be more prone to chronic headaches, including tension-type headaches and migraines.
- **Connection:** Shared mechanisms in the nervous system may contribute to the overlap between fibromyalgia and migraines.

Chronic Fatigue Syndrome (CFS)

- **Description:** CFS, also known as myalgic encephalomyelitis (ME), is characterized by persistent, unexplained fatigue that is not alleviated by rest.
- **Connection:** There is significant symptom overlap between fibromyalgia and CFS, and some individuals may be diagnosed with both conditions.

Depression and Anxiety

- **Description:** Mood disorders, such as depression and anxiety, are common among individuals with fibromyalgia.
- **Connection:** The chronic nature of fibromyalgia, coupled with the impact on daily life and function, can contribute to emotional distress.

Rheumatoid Arthritis (RA)

- **Description:** RA is an autoimmune disorder that primarily affects the joints, causing pain, swelling, and stiffness.

- **Connection:** While fibromyalgia is not an autoimmune disorder, individuals with RA may also experience fibromyalgia-like symptoms.

Osteoarthritis

- **Description:** Osteoarthritis is a degenerative joint condition that can cause pain and stiffness.
- **Connection:** Fibromyalgia and osteoarthritis can coexist, and distinguishing between the two conditions is important for effective management.

Temporomandibular Joint Disorders (TMJ)

- **Description:** TMJ disorders involve pain and dysfunction in the jaw joint and the muscles that control jaw movement.
- **Connection:** Jaw pain and TMJ issues are commonly reported by individuals with fibromyalgia.

Interstitial Cystitis (IC)

- **Description:** IC is a chronic condition characterized by bladder pain and urinary urgency.

Connection: Individuals with fibromyalgia may be at a higher risk of developing IC, and both conditions share some common symptoms.

Systemic Lupus Erythematosus (SLE)

- **Description:** SLE is an autoimmune disease that can affect various organs and tissues, causing inflammation and pain.
- **Connection:** Fibromyalgia-like symptoms can occur in individuals with SLE, and distinguishing between the two is important for appropriate management.

Endometriosis

- **Description:** Endometriosis is a condition in which tissue similar to the lining of the uterus grows outside the uterus, leading to pain and fertility issues.
- **Connection:** Women with fibromyalgia may have a higher prevalence of endometriosis, and managing both conditions requires a comprehensive approach.

It's important for healthcare providers to consider the presence of comorbid conditions when diagnosing and managing fibromyalgia. A holistic and multidisciplinary approach that addresses both fibromyalgia symptoms and comorbidities is often necessary for comprehensive care. If you have concerns about comorbid conditions or are experiencing symptoms beyond those typically associated with fibromyalgia, discuss them with your healthcare provider for a thorough evaluation and appropriate management.

RESEARCH AND DEVELOPMENTS

Here are some general areas of research and potential developments related to fibromyalgia:

Biomarkers and Diagnosis

Researchers are exploring potential biomarkers that could aid in the diagnosis of fibromyalgia. Identifying reliable biomarkers could improve diagnostic accuracy and help distinguish fibromyalgia from other conditions with similar symptoms.

Neurobiological and Genetic Studies

Studies are investigating the neurobiological and genetic factors associated with fibromyalgia. Understanding the underlying genetic and neurological mechanisms may provide insights into the development and progression of the condition.

Central Sensitization Mechanisms

Central sensitization, where the nervous system becomes hypersensitive to stimuli, is a key feature of fibromyalgia. Ongoing research aims to unravel the mechanisms of central sensitization, potentially leading to targeted treatments.

Pharmacological Research

Researchers are exploring new pharmacological approaches for treating fibromyalgia. This includes the development of medications that target specific pathways involved in pain processing and neurotransmitter regulation.

Non-Pharmacological Interventions

Continued research is focused on non-pharmacological interventions, such as cognitive-behavioral therapy (CBT), physical therapy, and exercise programs. Understanding the effectiveness of these interventions can contribute to improved treatment strategies.

Patient-Reported Outcomes

Studies are emphasizing patient-reported outcomes to better understand the impact of fibromyalgia on individuals' lives. This includes assessing quality of life, functional abilities, and the patient experience.

Digital Health and Telemedicine

The integration of digital health tools and telemedicine in fibromyalgia management is an area of growing interest. Mobile apps, wearable devices, and virtual healthcare platforms are being explored to enhance monitoring and support.

Collaborative Research Networks

Collaborative efforts among researchers and institutions are fostering a better understanding of fibromyalgia. Networks and consortia are working together to collect and analyze data on a larger scale.

Immunological Factors

Some studies are investigating the potential role of immunological factors in fibromyalgia. Understanding the immune system's involvement could lead to novel therapeutic approaches.

It's important to stay updated with the latest research findings through reputable medical journals and healthcare news sources. If you are interested in the most recent developments in fibromyalgia research, consider checking recent publications or consulting with healthcare professionals who specialize in the field. Keep in mind that research is an evolving field, and new insights may lead to advancements in our understanding and management of fibromyalgia.

COPING STRATEGIES

Coping with fibromyalgia involves a combination of medical management, lifestyle adjustments, and psychological strategies. Here are some coping strategies that individuals with fibromyalgia may find helpful:

Education and Self-awareness

- Learn about fibromyalgia to better understand the condition, its symptoms, and potential triggers.
- Keep a symptom journal to track patterns, identify triggers, and share information with healthcare providers.

Pacing Activities

- Break tasks into smaller, manageable segments to avoid overexertion.
- Prioritize activities and balance periods of activity with rest.

Regular Exercise

- Engage in low-impact exercises regularly, such as walking, swimming, or gentle yoga.

- Start with activities of short duration and low intensity, gradually increasing as tolerated.

Stress Management Techniques

- Practice stress-reducing techniques, including deep breathing, meditation, and progressive muscle relaxation.
- Identify and address sources of stress in daily life.

Quality Sleep

- Establish a consistent sleep routine and create a comfortable sleep environment.
- Practice good sleep hygiene, such as avoiding caffeine and electronic devices before bedtime.

Balanced Diet

- Maintain a well-balanced diet with a focus on nutrient-rich foods.
- Stay hydrated and consider consulting a registered dietitian for personalized dietary guidance.

Support System

- Build a support system of friends, family, and healthcare professionals.
- Join fibromyalgia support groups to connect with others who share similar experiences.

Cognitive-Behavioral Therapy (CBT)

- Consider CBT to address negative thought patterns and develop coping strategies.
- Learn techniques to manage stress, anxiety, and pain perception.

Occupational Therapy

- Consult with an occupational therapist for strategies to adapt daily activities and reduce strain on the body.
- Receive guidance on ergonomic adjustments in the home and workplace.

Mind-Body Practices

- Explore mind-body practices such as meditation, tai chi, or qigong to improve relaxation and mindfulness.

- Incorporate activities that promote mental and emotional well-being.

Hot and Cold Therapy

- Use heat packs or warm baths for muscle relaxation and pain relief.
- Cold packs can be applied to reduce inflammation and numb localized areas of pain.

Medication Management

- Work closely with healthcare providers to manage medications and adjust dosages as needed.
- Communicate openly about medication effectiveness and any side effects experienced.

Set Realistic Goals

- Establish achievable goals, both short-term and long-term.
- Celebrate small accomplishments and recognize personal achievements.

Creative Outlets

- Engage in creative activities, such as art, music, or writing, as a form of self-expression and stress relief.

Stay Informed

- Keep up-to-date with reputable sources of information on fibromyalgia.
- Advocate for yourself by being informed about your condition during healthcare discussions.

Individuals with fibromyalgia often benefit from a holistic and individualized approach to coping. It's important to consult with healthcare professionals, including rheumatologists, pain specialists, and mental health professionals, to develop a comprehensive management plan tailored to specific needs. Regular communication with the healthcare team helps ensure that coping strategies are effective and adjusted as necessary.

IMPACT ON QUALITY OF LIFE

Fibromyalgia can have a significant impact on various aspects of an individual's quality of life. The symptoms and challenges associated with this condition can affect physical, emotional, and social well-being. Here are some ways in which fibromyalgia may impact quality of life:

Pain and Discomfort

- **Constant Pain:** Widespread pain and discomfort can be persistent, affecting daily activities and reducing overall comfort.
- **Tender Points:** The presence of tender points can make certain movements or positions painful.

Fatigue and Sleep Disturbances

- **Chronic Fatigue:** Persistent fatigue can lead to a lack of energy and motivation.
- **Sleep Disruptions:** Difficulty falling asleep, staying asleep, or achieving restorative sleep can contribute to overall tiredness and exacerbate other symptoms.

Cognitive Challenges ("Fibro Fog")

- **Memory Issues:** Difficulty with concentration and memory can impact work, daily tasks, and overall cognitive function.
- **Mental Clarity:** "Fibro fog" can lead to a feeling of mental fogginess or confusion.

Impact on Mental Health

- **Depression and Anxiety:** Living with chronic pain and fatigue can contribute to feelings of sadness, frustration, and anxiety.
- **Social Isolation:** Challenges in participating in social activities and events may lead to feelings of isolation.

Physical Limitations

- **Reduced Mobility:** Pain and stiffness can limit physical activities, leading to a decrease in overall mobility.
- **Functional Impairments:** Fibromyalgia symptoms may impact the ability to perform certain tasks, both at home and at work.

Impact on Work and Employment

- **Reduced Work Productivity:** Absenteeism and presenteeism may occur due to the impact of symptoms on work performance.
- **Workplace Accommodations:** Some individuals may require accommodations to manage their condition effectively.

Financial Strain

- **Medical Expenses:** Ongoing medical appointments, treatments, and medications may contribute to financial strain.
- **Work-related Issues:** Difficulty maintaining employment or reduced work hours can affect income.

Impact on Relationships

- **Family Dynamics:** Fibromyalgia can affect family relationships due to changes in roles, responsibilities, and social activities.
- **Intimate Relationships:** Physical and emotional challenges may impact intimate relationships.

Emotional Well-being

- **Loss of Independence:** The need for support and assistance may challenge one's sense of independence.
- **Emotional Resilience:** Coping with a chronic condition may require ongoing emotional resilience.

Treatment Side Effects

- **Medication Side Effects:** Some medications used to manage fibromyalgia symptoms may have side effects that impact overall well-being.
- **Adverse Reactions:** Individuals may experience adverse reactions to certain treatments or interventions.

Despite these challenges, it's important to note that with proper management, support, and coping strategies, individuals with fibromyalgia can lead fulfilling lives. A multidisciplinary approach involving healthcare professionals, support networks, and self-care can help mitigate the impact of fibromyalgia on quality of life. Additionally, ongoing research and advancements in treatment may offer new strategies for improving outcomes and addressing the various aspects of well-being affected by fibromyalgia.

PEDIATRIC FIBROMYALGIA

Pediatric fibromyalgia is a condition that affects children and adolescents and shares similarities with fibromyalgia in adults. However, there are some differences in terms of symptom presentation, diagnosis, and management in the pediatric population. Here are key points related to pediatric fibromyalgia:

Symptoms

- **Pain:** Children with fibromyalgia experience widespread pain similar to adults. However, they may have difficulty expressing the location and nature of their pain.

- **Fatigue:** Chronic fatigue is a common symptom, impacting energy levels and daily functioning.

- **Sleep Disturbances:** Sleep disruptions, such as difficulty falling asleep and staying asleep, may be present.

Diagnosis

- **Challenges in Diagnosis:** Diagnosing fibromyalgia in children can be challenging due to the overlap of symptoms with other pediatric conditions.

- **Similar Criteria:** Diagnosis may follow criteria similar to those used in adults, but pediatric-specific criteria have also been proposed.

Common Comorbidities

- **Headaches:** Children with fibromyalgia often experience tension headaches or migraines.
- **Gastrointestinal Issues:** Some may have comorbid conditions like irritable bowel syndrome (IBS).

Impact on Daily Life

- School Performance: Fibromyalgia symptoms can affect a child's ability to concentrate and participate in school activities.
- Social Functioning: Chronic pain and fatigue may impact a child's social life and extracurricular activities.

Psychological Factors

- **Emotional Impact:** Children with fibromyalgia may experience emotional challenges, including mood swings, anxiety, and depression.
- **Cognitive Functioning:** "Fibro fog" can affect cognitive functioning in school and daily life.

Treatment Approaches

- **Multidisciplinary Care:** Similar to adults, a multidisciplinary approach is often used in pediatric fibromyalgia management. This may include pediatric rheumatologists, pain specialists, physical therapists, and psychologists.
- **Cognitive-Behavioral Therapy (CBT):** CBT can help children and adolescents develop coping strategies for pain and stress.
- **Physical Therapy:** Tailored exercise programs and physical therapy can improve flexibility and reduce pain.
- **Medication:** Medications such as pain relievers and antidepressants may be considered, with careful monitoring of dosage and side effects.

Family Support

- **Educating Families:** Providing education to parents and caregivers about fibromyalgia is crucial for understanding and managing the condition in a pediatric setting.
- **Creating Supportive Environments:** Creating supportive environments at home and in school is essential for the well-being of the child.

Long-Term Outlook

- **Variable Course:** The course of pediatric fibromyalgia can be variable, and symptoms may improve or persist into adulthood.

- **Transition to Adult Care:** As children with fibromyalgia transition to adulthood, they may need ongoing support in managing their condition.

Early intervention, a supportive environment, and a comprehensive treatment plan can contribute to better outcomes for children and adolescents with fibromyalgia. Pediatric rheumatologists and healthcare professionals experienced in treating pediatric pain conditions play a critical role in the diagnosis and management of pediatric fibromyalgia. If there are concerns about a child's symptoms, it's important to seek evaluation and guidance from healthcare professionals familiar with pediatric rheumatology.

MEDICATIONS

The management of fibromyalgia often involves a combination of medications, lifestyle modifications, and other therapeutic approaches. It's important to note that there is no cure for fibromyalgia, and treatment aims to alleviate symptoms and improve the overall quality of life. The choice of medications may vary based on individual symptoms and response. Here are some medications commonly used in the management of fibromyalgia:

Analgesics (Pain Relievers)

- **Acetaminophen:** It can help reduce pain but does not have anti-inflammatory properties. It's generally considered a first-line treatment.

- **Nonsteroidal Anti-Inflammatory Drugs (NSAIDs):** Drugs like ibuprofen or naproxen can help with pain and inflammation, but they may be less effective for fibromyalgia-related pain.

Antidepressants

- **Tricyclic Antidepressants (TCAs):** Amitriptyline and nortriptyline are TCAs that may help alleviate pain, improve sleep, and reduce fatigue. They are often used at lower doses than those used for depression.

- **Selective Serotonin Reuptake Inhibitors (SSRIs):** Fluoxetine and duloxetine are SSRIs that may be prescribed to help manage pain and improve mood.

- **Serotonin-Norepinephrine Reuptake Inhibitors (SNRIs):** Duloxetine (Cymbalta) is an SNRI that has been FDA-approved for the treatment of fibromyalgia. It can help with pain, fatigue, and mood.

Anticonvulsants

- **Pregabalin (Lyrica):** Pregabalin is an anticonvulsant that has been approved for the treatment of fibromyalgia. It can help reduce pain and improve sleep.

- **Gabapentin:** Similar to pregabalin, gabapentin may be prescribed to help manage pain and improve sleep.

Muscle Relaxants

- **Cyclobenzaprine:** This muscle relaxant can help alleviate muscle spasms and improve sleep. It is often used in the short term due to potential side effects.

Opioid Medications

- **Opioids:** Opioid medications may be prescribed in some cases for the management of severe pain. However, they are generally not considered first-line due to concerns about dependence and other side effects.

Sleep Medications

- **Sedative-Hypnotics:** Medications such as zolpidem (Ambien) or trazodone may be prescribed to improve sleep in individuals with fibromyalgia.

It's crucial for individuals with fibromyalgia to work closely with their healthcare providers to determine the most appropriate medications based on their specific symptoms, medical history, and potential side effects. Additionally, a multidisciplinary approach that includes lifestyle modifications, physical therapy, and psychological support is often recommended for comprehensive fibromyalgia management.

It's important to note that medication management should be closely monitored, and adjustments may be made over time to address changes in symptoms or the development of potential side effects. Regular communication with healthcare providers is key to optimizing treatment and improving overall well-being.

PHYSICAL THERAPY

Physical therapy is a crucial component of the comprehensive management of fibromyalgia. A physical therapist (PT) can work with individuals to address specific musculoskeletal issues, improve flexibility and strength, and develop strategies to manage pain. The goals of physical therapy for fibromyalgia include enhancing functional abilities, reducing pain, and improving overall quality of life. Here are key aspects of physical therapy for fibromyalgia:

Individualized Assessment

A physical therapist will conduct a thorough assessment of the individual's physical condition, taking into account pain levels, joint mobility, muscle strength, and any areas of tenderness.

Exercise Programs

- **Aerobic Exercise:** Low-impact aerobic exercises, such as walking, swimming, or stationary cycling, can help improve cardiovascular fitness and reduce overall pain.
- **Strength Training:** Targeted strength training exercises, tailored to the individual's abilities, can enhance muscle strength and support joint function.

Flexibility Exercises: Stretching and flexibility exercises can improve joint range of motion and reduce stiffness.

Pain Management Techniques

- PTs may teach individuals pain management techniques, including positioning, relaxation exercises, and gentle massage.
- Modalities such as heat or cold therapy may be incorporated to help alleviate pain and muscle stiffness.

Posture and Body Mechanics

- Education on proper posture and body mechanics is important to prevent strain on muscles and joints during daily activities.
- PTs can provide guidance on ergonomic adjustments at home and in the workplace.

Activity Pacing

- Teaching individuals how to pace their activities to avoid overexertion and prevent flare-ups is a key aspect of physical therapy.

- Breaking tasks into manageable segments and incorporating rest breaks are strategies often recommended.

Education and Self-Management

- PTs can provide education about fibromyalgia, helping individuals understand their condition and empowering them to actively participate in their own care.
- Self-management strategies, including home exercises and lifestyle modifications, are often emphasized.

Assistive Devices and Adaptive Equipment

- If necessary, physical therapists can assess the need for assistive devices or adaptive equipment to enhance mobility and independence.

Functional Capacity Evaluation

- Evaluating functional capacity helps determine an individual's ability to perform daily activities and provides insights for setting realistic goals.

Collaboration with Other Healthcare Providers

Physical therapists often collaborate with other members of the healthcare team, including rheumatologists, pain specialists, and occupational therapists, to provide comprehensive care.

Home Exercise Programs

Providing individuals with tailored home exercise programs allows them to continue therapeutic exercises independently between physical therapy sessions.

It's important for individuals with fibromyalgia to communicate openly with their physical therapist about their symptoms, preferences, and any concerns. Physical therapy is typically part of a multidisciplinary approach that may also include medication management, cognitive-behavioral therapy, and lifestyle modifications. Regular follow-up sessions with a physical therapist can help track progress, modify treatment plans as needed, and provide ongoing support for managing fibromyalgia symptoms.

EXERCISE PROGRAMS

Exercise is a crucial component of managing fibromyalgia symptoms. Engaging in a regular and tailored exercise program can help improve muscle strength, flexibility, and overall well-being. However, it's essential to approach exercise for fibromyalgia cautiously, considering individual limitations and preferences.

Here are some key considerations for developing an exercise program for individuals with fibromyalgia:

Low-Impact Aerobic Exercise

- **Walking:** A low-impact activity like walking is often well-tolerated and can be easily incorporated into a daily routine.

- **Swimming or Water Aerobics:** The buoyancy of water reduces impact on joints, making aquatic exercises an excellent option.

- **Cycling:** Stationary or outdoor cycling can provide cardiovascular benefits with minimal impact on joints.

Strength Training

- **Light Weights:** Start with light weights and gradually increase resistance as tolerated. Resistance bands are also effective.
- **Bodyweight Exercises:** Exercises that use the body's own resistance, such as squats or lunges, can be adapted to individual fitness levels.

Flexibility and Stretching

- **Gentle Stretching:** Incorporate gentle stretching exercises to improve flexibility and reduce muscle stiffness.
- **Yoga or Tai Chi:** These mind-body practices combine gentle movements with deep breathing and can enhance flexibility, balance, and relaxation.

Pacing Activities

- **Break Tasks:** Divide tasks into smaller, manageable segments, and take breaks to avoid overexertion.
- **Gradual Progression:** Start with shorter durations and lower intensities, gradually increasing as tolerance improves.

Warm-Up and Cool Down

- **Warm-Up:** Begin each session with a 5-10 minute warm-up, such as light aerobic activity or gentle stretching.
- **Cool Down:** End with a cool-down, including stretching exercises to prevent muscle stiffness.

Mind-Body Practices

- **Meditation and Relaxation:** Incorporate mindfulness meditation or relaxation techniques to manage stress and improve overall well-being.
- **Breathing Exercises:** Focused breathing exercises can help promote relaxation and reduce anxiety.

Individualized Approach

- **Consult a Professional:** Before starting an exercise program, consult with a healthcare professional or a physical therapist familiar with fibromyalgia.
- **Tailored Programs:** Work with a fitness professional who understands fibromyalgia to design a personalized exercise program.

Regular Routine

- **Consistency is Key:** Establishing a regular exercise routine is important for long-term benefits.
- **Listen to Your Body:** Pay attention to how your body responds to different exercises, and adjust intensity and duration accordingly.

Social Support

- **Exercise with Others:** Engaging in group activities or classes can provide social support and motivation.
- **Supportive Environment:** Create an exercise environment that feels comfortable and supportive.

Adaptability

- **Modify as Needed:** Be willing to modify your exercise routine based on fluctuations in symptoms or energy levels.
- **Choose Enjoyable Activities:** Select activities that you enjoy to make exercise more enjoyable and sustainable.

It's crucial to note that individuals with fibromyalgia may have varying levels of fitness and different tolerances for exercise. The key is to start slowly, gradually increase intensity, and listen to the body. If there are concerns or uncertainties about starting an exercise program, it's advisable to seek guidance from a healthcare professional or a qualified fitness expert familiar with fibromyalgia.

COGNITIVE-BEHAVIORAL THERAPY (CBT)

Cognitive-Behavioral Therapy (CBT) is a therapeutic approach that has been found to be effective in managing various mental health conditions, including fibromyalgia. CBT for fibromyalgia focuses on addressing the interplay between thoughts, feelings, and behaviors, with the goal of promoting positive changes in how individuals perceive and cope with their symptoms. Here are key components of CBT for fibromyalgia:

Cognitive Restructuring

- **Identifying Negative Thoughts:** Individuals work with a therapist to identify and challenge negative or unhelpful thoughts related to their pain and symptoms.
- **Changing Thought Patterns:** Through cognitive restructuring, individuals learn to replace negative thought patterns with more realistic and positive thoughts.

Behavioral Activation

- **Activity Pacing:** CBT often involves teaching individuals how to pace their activities to avoid overexertion and prevent exacerbation of symptoms.

- **Goal Setting:** Collaboratively setting realistic and achievable goals helps individuals regain a sense of control over their lives.

Stress Management

- **Relaxation Techniques:** Learning and practicing relaxation techniques, such as deep breathing, progressive muscle relaxation, or guided imagery, can help manage stress and reduce muscle tension.
- **Stress Reduction Strategies:** Identifying and addressing sources of stress in daily life is an integral part of CBT for fibromyalgia.

Pain Coping Skills

- **Developing Coping Strategies:** Individuals learn adaptive coping strategies to manage pain, such as mindfulness, distraction techniques, or positive imagery.
- **Problem-Solving:** Developing problem-solving skills helps individuals address challenges related to their symptoms.

Activity and Sleep Regulation

- **Establishing Routines:** Creating and maintaining regular routines for activities and sleep promotes better overall functioning.

- **Sleep Hygiene:** CBT often includes education on improving sleep hygiene and addressing factors contributing to sleep disturbances.

Education and Psychoeducation

- **Understanding Fibromyalgia:** CBT includes psychoeducation to enhance individuals' understanding of fibromyalgia and its impact on physical and emotional well-being.

- **Promoting Self-Help:** Individuals are empowered to become active participants in their own care and develop skills for self-management.

Graded Exposure

- **Gradual Exposure:** Graded exposure involves gradually facing and overcoming activities or situations that may have been avoided due to fear of pain or discomfort.

- **Building Confidence:** Successive approximations help build confidence and reduce avoidance behaviors.

Mindfulness-Based Approaches

- **Mindfulness Meditation:** Mindfulness techniques, including meditation and mindful awareness, are integrated into CBT to promote present-moment focus and acceptance.
- **Mind-Body Integration:** Combining cognitive and mindfulness strategies helps individuals develop a holistic approach to managing their symptoms.

Therapeutic Relationship

- **Collaboration:** CBT is a collaborative process, and the therapeutic relationship between the individual and the therapist is crucial.
- **Feedback and Support:** Regular feedback and support from the therapist facilitate the learning and application of coping skills.

CBT for fibromyalgia is typically conducted in individual or group settings and may involve a set number of sessions. It's important to work with a mental health professional trained in

CBT and experienced in addressing the specific challenges associated with fibromyalgia. The skills learned in CBT can have lasting benefits, helping individuals better cope with their symptoms and improve their overall quality of life.

SUPPORT GROUPS

Support groups can play a valuable role in the overall management of fibromyalgia by providing individuals with a platform to share experiences, gain insights, and receive emotional support. Connecting with others who understand the challenges of living with fibromyalgia can be empowering and contribute to a sense of community. Here are some key aspects of fibromyalgia support groups:

Shared Understanding

Support groups bring together individuals who share a common experience of living with fibromyalgia. This shared understanding fosters empathy and a sense of validation.

Emotional Support

Dealing with chronic pain and the impact of fibromyalgia on daily life can be emotionally challenging. Support groups offer a safe space to express feelings, share concerns, and receive emotional support from others who can relate.

Information Exchange

Members of support groups often exchange practical information, coping strategies, and tips for managing symptoms. This information-sharing can be particularly beneficial for those newly diagnosed or exploring new approaches to symptom management.

Education

Support groups may invite healthcare professionals to provide educational sessions on various aspects of fibromyalgia, including treatment options, lifestyle modifications, and coping strategies. This helps members stay informed and empowered in managing their condition.

Coping Strategies

Members can discuss and share personal coping strategies that have proven effective for them. This may include approaches to managing pain, improving sleep, and enhancing overall well-being.

Reducing Isolation

Fibromyalgia can sometimes lead to feelings of isolation. Support groups provide an opportunity to connect with others who face similar challenges, reducing the sense of isolation and fostering a supportive community.

Advocacy and Empowerment

Support groups can empower individuals to become advocates for themselves and others with fibromyalgia. Advocacy efforts may include raising awareness, promoting research, and addressing issues related to healthcare access and understanding.

Online and In-Person Options

Support groups may take various forms, including in-person meetings, telephone conferences, or online forums. Online options can be particularly convenient for individuals who may face mobility challenges or live in remote areas.

Peer-Led and Professionally Facilitated Groups

Some support groups are peer-led, where individuals with fibromyalgia take on leadership roles. Others may be professionally facilitated, with a healthcare professional guiding discussions and providing expertise.

Building Resilience

Sharing stories of resilience and personal growth can inspire others in the group. Hearing about others' journeys towards acceptance and a meaningful life despite fibromyalgia can be motivating.

Positive Social Interaction

Support groups offer an opportunity for positive social interaction. Building connections with others who understand the challenges can contribute to a sense of belonging and well-being.

It's important to find a support group that aligns with individual preferences and needs. Some individuals may prefer in-person meetings, while others may find online forums or telephone conferences more accessible. Healthcare providers, local community centers, or national fibromyalgia organizations may be able to provide information about available support groups.

Remember that participation in a support group is voluntary, and individuals can choose the level of involvement that feels comfortable for them. Additionally, support groups are just one aspect of a comprehensive approach to managing fibromyalgia, which may also include medical treatment, lifestyle adjustments, and other forms of support.

IMPACT ON MENTAL HEALTH

Fibromyalgia can have a significant impact on mental health due to the chronic nature of the condition, its associated symptoms, and the challenges individuals face in managing their health. Here are ways in which fibromyalgia may affect mental health:

Chronic Pain and Discomfort

- **Emotional Toll:** Living with persistent pain and discomfort can lead to emotional distress, frustration, and a sense of helplessness.
- **Psychological Impact:** Chronic pain conditions are often associated with an increased risk of anxiety and depression.

Fatigue and Sleep Disturbances

- **Cognitive Functioning:** Chronic fatigue can affect cognitive functioning, leading to difficulties with memory, concentration, and overall mental clarity.
- **Mood Disturbances:** Sleep disturbances can contribute to mood disorders, including irritability, mood swings, and feelings of exhaustion.

Cognitive Dysfunction ("Fibro Fog")

- **Memory Issues:** Fibromyalgia is often associated with cognitive dysfunction, commonly referred to as "fibro fog." This can include difficulties with memory, attention, and processing information.

- **Impact on Daily Functioning:** Cognitive challenges can affect performance at work or school and contribute to feelings of frustration and stress.

Emotional Well-being

- **Anxiety:** The uncertainty of living with a chronic condition and the impact on daily life can contribute to anxiety.

- **Depression:** The persistent nature of fibromyalgia symptoms, coupled with the challenges of managing the condition, may increase the risk of depression.

Social Isolation

- **Reduced Social Participation:** Individuals with fibromyalgia may experience limitations in participating in social activities due to pain, fatigue, or other symptoms.

- **Impact on Relationships:** Social isolation can contribute to feelings of loneliness and may impact relationships with family and friends.

Impact on Self-Esteem

- **Functional Limitations:** Physical limitations and the need for accommodations can impact an individual's sense of independence and self-worth.
- **Adjustment to New Realities:** Adjusting to life with fibromyalgia may involve adapting to a new set of capabilities and limitations, which can influence self-esteem.

Stress and Coping

- **Daily Stressors:** Managing the demands of daily life alongside fibromyalgia symptoms can be stressful.
- **Coping Strategies:** Individuals may need to develop and adapt coping strategies to deal with stressors effectively.

Impact on Work and Employment

- **Work-related Stress:** The impact of fibromyalgia on work performance, absenteeism, and workplace relationships can contribute to stress.

- **Financial Concerns:** Difficulty maintaining employment or reducing work hours may lead to financial strain.

It's important to recognize the interconnectedness of physical and mental health in individuals with fibromyalgia. Addressing mental health concerns is a vital aspect of comprehensive fibromyalgia management. Multidisciplinary approaches, including medical treatment, cognitive-behavioral therapy, support groups, and lifestyle adjustments, can contribute to improved mental well-being.

Individuals experiencing mental health challenges related to fibromyalgia are encouraged to seek support from healthcare professionals, including mental health providers, who can offer tailored interventions and support. Open communication with healthcare providers, family, and friends is crucial for building a strong support network and addressing both the physical and emotional aspects of living with fibromyalgia.

PEDIATRIC FIBROMYALGIA

Pediatric fibromyalgia is a condition characterized by widespread musculoskeletal pain, fatigue, and other symptoms similar to those seen in adults with fibromyalgia. While fibromyalgia is more commonly diagnosed in adults, it can also affect children and adolescents. Here are key points related to pediatric fibromyalgia:

Symptoms

- **Pain:** Children with fibromyalgia experience chronic pain, often described as aching or stiffness, in multiple areas of the body.
- **Fatigue:** Persistent fatigue is a common symptom, impacting energy levels and daily functioning.
- **Sleep Disturbances:** Similar to adults, children with fibromyalgia may experience difficulties falling asleep, staying asleep, or achieving restorative sleep.

Diagnosis

- **Challenges in Diagnosis:** Diagnosing fibromyalgia in children can be challenging due to the overlap of symptoms with other pediatric conditions.

- **Diagnostic Criteria:** Pediatric fibromyalgia may be diagnosed using criteria similar to those applied in adults, but there are also pediatric-specific criteria.

Common Comorbidities

- **Headaches:** Children with fibromyalgia often experience tension headaches or migraines.
- **Gastrointestinal Issues:** Some may have comorbid conditions like irritable bowel syndrome (IBS).

Impact on Daily Life

- **School Performance:** Fibromyalgia symptoms can affect a child's ability to concentrate and participate in school activities.
- **Social Functioning:** Chronic pain and fatigue may impact a child's social life and extracurricular activities.

Psychological Factors

- **Emotional Impact:** Children with fibromyalgia may experience emotional challenges, including mood swings, anxiety, and depression.

- **Cognitive Functioning:** "Fibro fog," characterized by cognitive difficulties, can affect academic performance and daily activities.

Treatment Approaches

- **Multidisciplinary Care:** Similar to adults, pediatric fibromyalgia management often involves a multidisciplinary approach. This may include pediatric rheumatologists, pain specialists, physical therapists, and psychologists.
- **Cognitive-Behavioral Therapy (CBT):** CBT can help children and adolescents develop coping strategies for pain and stress.
- **Physical Therapy:** Tailored exercise programs and physical therapy can improve flexibility and reduce pain.
- **Medication:** Medications such as pain relievers and antidepressants may be considered, with careful monitoring of dosage and side effects.

Family Support

- **Educating Families:** Providing education to parents and caregivers about fibromyalgia is crucial for understanding and managing the condition in a pediatric setting.

Creating Supportive Environments: Creating supportive environments at home and in school is essential for the well-being of the child.

Long-Term Outlook

- **Variable Course:** The course of pediatric fibromyalgia can be variable, and symptoms may improve or persist into adulthood.
- **Transition to Adult Care:** As children with fibromyalgia transition to adulthood, they may need ongoing support in managing their condition.

Early intervention, a supportive environment, and a comprehensive treatment plan can contribute to better outcomes for children and adolescents with fibromyalgia. Pediatric rheumatologists and healthcare professionals experienced in treating pediatric pain conditions play a critical role in the diagnosis and management of pediatric fibromyalgia. If there are concerns about a child's symptoms, it's important to seek evaluation and guidance from healthcare professionals familiar with pediatric rheumatology.

RESEARCH AND DEVELOPMENTS

Here are some areas of research and potential developments in fibromyalgia:

Biological Mechanisms

Research is focused on understanding the biological and neurological mechanisms that contribute to the development and maintenance of fibromyalgia. This includes investigations into central sensitization, neurotransmitter imbalances, and the role of the immune system.

Genetic Studies

Studies examining the genetic factors associated with fibromyalgia aim to identify specific genes or genetic markers that may contribute to an individual's susceptibility to the condition. This research may provide insights into potential risk factors and personalized treatment approaches.

Neuroimaging Studies

Advances in neuroimaging techniques, such as functional magnetic resonance imaging (fMRI) and positron emission tomography (PET), are being used to explore brain changes and abnormalities in individuals with fibromyalgia. These studies may contribute to a better understanding of pain processing in the central nervous system.

Biomarkers

Identification of reliable biomarkers for fibromyalgia is an area of active research. Biomarkers could aid in diagnosis, treatment selection, and monitoring disease progression. Various potential biomarkers, including cytokines and neurochemicals, are being investigated.

New Medications

Clinical trials are ongoing to evaluate the efficacy and safety of new medications for fibromyalgia. This includes drugs targeting specific pathways involved in pain modulation, neurotransmitter regulation, and inflammation.

Non-Pharmacological Interventions

Research continues to explore the effectiveness of non-pharmacological interventions, such as different forms of exercise, cognitive-behavioral therapy, mindfulness-based approaches, and complementary therapies like acupuncture.

Understanding the most beneficial combinations of treatments is an active area of investigation.

Patient Subgroups

Researchers are exploring the concept of patient subgroups within the broader category of fibromyalgia. Identifying distinct subtypes of fibromyalgia based on symptom patterns, genetic factors, or other characteristics may lead to more targeted and personalized treatment strategies.

Digital Health and Telemedicine

The use of digital health tools and telemedicine in fibromyalgia management is an evolving area. Mobile applications, wearable devices, and virtual care platforms are being studied for their potential to support self-management and improve communication between patients and healthcare providers.

Impact of Microbiome

Some studies are investigating the role of the gut microbiome in fibromyalgia. Emerging evidence suggests a potential link between gut health, inflammation, and fibromyalgia symptoms.

Educational Initiatives

Efforts are being made to increase awareness and understanding of fibromyalgia among healthcare providers and the general public. This includes educational initiatives to improve the recognition and appropriate management of the condition.

It's essential to stay updated on the latest research findings through reputable sources, medical journals, and healthcare providers. Participation in clinical trials, when appropriate, can also contribute to the advancement of fibromyalgia research and the development of new treatment options.

WORKPLACE ACCOMMODATIONS

Individuals with fibromyalgia may face challenges in the workplace due to symptoms such as chronic pain, fatigue, and cognitive difficulties. Workplace accommodations can play a crucial role in helping employees with fibromyalgia manage their condition and maintain productivity. Accommodations are often tailored to the individual's specific needs and may involve modifications to the work environment or adjustments to job responsibilities. Here are some examples of workplace accommodations for individuals with fibromyalgia:

Flexible Work Hours

- **Flexible Scheduling:** Allow flexibility in work hours, such as adjusted start and end times, to accommodate variations in energy levels and symptom severity.
- **Part-Time or Reduced Hours:** Consider offering part-time or reduced hours for individuals who may need more frequent breaks or shorter workdays.

Telecommuting and Remote Work

- **Remote Work Options:** Provide the opportunity for telecommuting or remote work to reduce the impact of commuting and create a more comfortable work environment.

- **Flexible Location:** Allow flexibility in the location of work, enabling employees to work from home or other suitable environments.

Ergonomic Adjustments

- **Ergonomic Workspace:** Modify workstations to be ergonomically friendly, including adjustable chairs, keyboards, and monitors to reduce physical strain.
- **Sit-Stand Desks:** Offer sit-stand desks to allow employees to change positions throughout the day and reduce the impact of prolonged sitting.

Job Task Modifications

- **Job Rotation:** Implement job rotation or task-sharing to minimize repetitive tasks and prevent overexertion.
- **Breaking Tasks into Smaller Units:** Break down complex tasks into smaller, more manageable units to accommodate reduced concentration and fatigue.

Assistive Technology

- **Speech-to-Text Software:** Provide speech-to-text software or other assistive technologies to support individuals with cognitive difficulties or pain-related typing challenges.
- **Ergonomic Accessories:** Offer ergonomic accessories such as trackballs, ergonomic mice, and voice-activated tools.

Quiet or Rest Areas

- **Quiet Spaces:** Designate quiet areas or rest spaces where employees can take short breaks to manage symptoms or rest when needed.
- **Flexible Breaks:** Allow flexibility in break times to accommodate the need for rest and relaxation.

Supportive Chairs and Seating

Specialized Seating: Provide supportive chairs or seating options that reduce pressure on sensitive areas and improve overall comfort.

Education and Awareness

- **Training for Colleagues:** Conduct training sessions to raise awareness among colleagues about fibromyalgia, its symptoms, and the importance of creating a supportive work environment.
- **Supervisor Education:** Train supervisors and managers on how to recognize and support employees with fibromyalgia.

Job Coaching and Mentoring

- **Job Coaching:** Offer job coaching or mentoring to help employees navigate their roles, set realistic goals, and develop effective coping strategies.
- **Performance Feedback:** Provide regular and constructive performance feedback to ensure ongoing support and communication.

Flexible Leave Policies

- **Sick Leave and Absence Policies:** Implement flexible sick leave policies to accommodate intermittent absences or flare-ups.

- **Medical Leave:** Offer extended medical leave when necessary, with clear communication about the process and return-to-work plans.

It's important for employers to engage in an interactive process with employees to determine the most effective accommodations for their specific needs. This process involves open communication, collaboration, and a willingness to make adjustments based on the individual's requirements. Additionally, accommodations should be periodically reviewed and modified as needed to ensure continued effectiveness.

QUALITY OF LIFE CONSIDERATIONS

Fibromyalgia can have a significant impact on various aspects of an individual's life, affecting not only physical health but also emotional well-being and overall quality of life. Quality of life considerations for individuals with fibromyalgia encompass a range of factors that influence daily functioning and overall satisfaction. Here are key aspects to consider:

Physical Health

- **Pain Management:** Effective pain management strategies, including medications, physical therapy, and lifestyle modifications, are crucial for improving physical well-being.

- **Fatigue Management:** Addressing fatigue through proper rest, sleep hygiene, and energy conservation techniques can contribute to better overall functioning.

Emotional Well-being

- **Mental Health Support:** Access to mental health resources, including counseling or therapy, can help individuals cope with the emotional challenges associated with fibromyalgia.

- **Stress Reduction:** Stress management techniques, such as mindfulness, relaxation exercises, and stress-reducing activities, can positively impact emotional well-being.

Social Relationships

- **Communication:** Open communication with family, friends, and colleagues about the challenges of living with fibromyalgia can foster understanding and support.
- **Social Support:** Building and maintaining a strong social support network is essential for emotional resilience and improved quality of life.

Occupational Considerations

- **Workplace Accommodations:** Tailoring the work environment, responsibilities, and schedules to accommodate the needs of individuals with fibromyalgia can contribute to job satisfaction and performance.
- **Career Planning:** Collaborative career planning that takes into account individual abilities, limitations, and goals helps individuals navigate their professional paths effectively.

Cognitive Functioning

- **Cognitive-Behavioral Strategies:** Implementing cognitive-behavioral strategies, including cognitive restructuring and mindfulness, can enhance cognitive functioning and mitigate "fibro fog."

- **Workspace Adaptations:** Making adaptations to the work or home environment, such as using assistive technology, can support cognitive functioning.

Physical Activity and Exercise

- **Tailored Exercise Programs:** Engaging in regular, low-impact exercise programs designed to accommodate individual abilities can improve physical fitness and overall well-being.

- **Balance and Flexibility:** Incorporating activities that enhance balance, flexibility, and strength can contribute to better physical health.

Sleep Quality

- **Sleep Hygiene:** Adopting good sleep hygiene practices, such as maintaining a consistent sleep schedule and creating a comfortable sleep environment, is crucial for managing fibromyalgia symptoms.

- **Sleep Interventions:** Discussing sleep-related issues with healthcare providers and exploring interventions, such as cognitive-behavioral therapy for insomnia (CBT-I), may be beneficial.

Nutrition and Lifestyle

- **Balanced Nutrition:** Adopting a balanced and nutritious diet can support overall health and energy levels.
- **Lifestyle Modifications:** Making appropriate lifestyle adjustments, such as managing stress, avoiding overexertion, and incorporating relaxation techniques, can positively impact quality of life.

Pacing and Goal Setting

- **Activity Pacing:** Learning to pace activities and set realistic goals helps individuals manage their energy levels and prevent overexertion.
- **Achievable Goals:** Setting achievable short-term and long-term goals contributes to a sense of accomplishment and empowerment.

Patient Education

- **Understanding Fibromyalgia:** Education about fibromyalgia, its symptoms, and available management strategies is empowering and helps individuals make informed decisions about their care.

- **Advocacy:** Encouraging self-advocacy and providing resources for individuals to navigate healthcare systems and access appropriate support.

Quality of life considerations for individuals with fibromyalgia are highly individualized, and a multidisciplinary approach involving healthcare professionals, social support networks, and self-management strategies is typically beneficial. Regular communication with healthcare providers, ongoing adaptation of coping strategies, and a proactive approach to managing symptoms contribute to an improved quality of life for individuals living with fibromyalgia.

CONCLUSION

Fibromyalgia is a complex and often challenging condition characterized by widespread musculoskeletal pain, fatigue, sleep disturbances, and various other symptoms. Its precise cause remains unclear, and the diagnosis is based on a combination of clinical symptoms, medical history, and exclusion of other conditions. Fibromyalgia significantly impacts the physical and mental well-being of individuals, affecting various aspects of daily life.

Managing fibromyalgia requires a comprehensive and individualized approach, often involving a multidisciplinary team of healthcare professionals. Treatment options may include medications, physical therapy, cognitive-behavioral therapy, and lifestyle modifications. The importance of a strong support system, including understanding and supportive healthcare providers, family, and friends, cannot be overstated.

It's essential for individuals with fibromyalgia to actively participate in their care, advocate for their needs, and explore a combination of strategies to improve their quality of life. Lifestyle adjustments, including regular exercise, stress management, and adequate sleep, can play a crucial role in symptom management.

Research and developments in fibromyalgia continue, exploring areas such as genetic factors, neurobiological mechanisms, and innovative treatment approaches. As our understanding of fibromyalgia evolves, ongoing efforts are directed toward improving diagnostic accuracy, developing targeted therapies, and enhancing the overall well-being of those affected by this condition.

While fibromyalgia poses significant challenges, advances in medical knowledge and increased awareness contribute to better support and management strategies for individuals living with this condition. Continued research, education, and advocacy are essential components of the ongoing effort to improve the lives of individuals with fibromyalgia. If you or someone you know is experiencing symptoms suggestive of fibromyalgia, seeking timely medical evaluation and support is crucial for accurate diagnosis and effective management.

www.ingramcontent.com/pod-product-compliance
Lightning Source LLC
Chambersburg PA
CBHW070914260726
48661CB00004B/1726